Lose 30 pounds fast by intermittent fasting

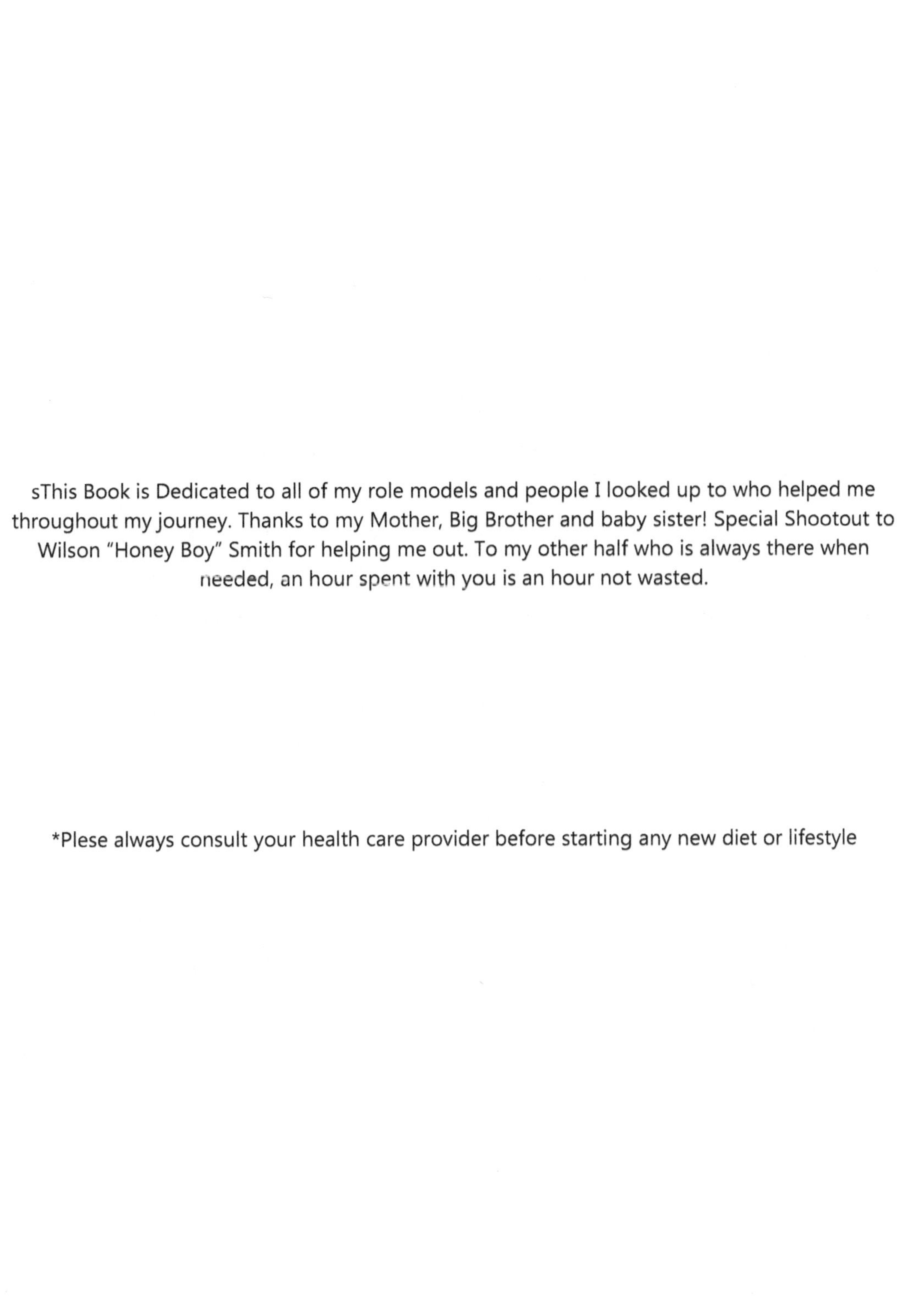

sThis Book is Dedicated to all of my role models and people I looked up to who helped me throughout my journey. Thanks to my Mother, Big Brother and baby sister! Special Shootout to Wilson "Honey Boy" Smith for helping me out. To my other half who is always there when needed, an hour spent with you is an hour not wasted.

*Plese always consult your health care provider before starting any new diet or lifestyle

INTRODUCTION

With so many diet trends out there, it is hard to determine which one to try. Many of us spend more time on many diet programs that we actually gain most of the weight back thus counteracting our desired results. Fasting may or may not be tried by many of us.

When we do try this type of dieting, we don't usually do this correctly or become frustrated by the restrictions that we give up. We end up feeling as though we wasted our time, effort and energy only to end up empty handed with the results.

Intermittent fasting is not something many have heard about. This is due to the fact that it is a fairly new way of eating. I am sure this new form of eating is soon to sweep the nation with benefits we could all enjoy. With this diet, one can be expected to not only lose weight but you could possibly live longer as well.

When this diet is done properly, your body can become better equipped to deal with the health conditions it may or not face in the future. This diet is very simple and the rewards are nothing but amazing. You will lose weight, burn that stubborn fat, hold on to lean muscle and even boost your growth hormone. After all that time you spent trying the latest fads, why not give this a try?

There are no restrictions with what you are able to eat while on the Intermittent Fasting Diet. Yep, reach for that greasy hamburger or fattening fries. The great thing about this lifestyle is that you can start your intermittent fasting anytime. As long as you go 16 hours without food with the exception of drinking water, tea, or black coffee. Continue this cycle daily and that's it. This eat stop eating method of dieting is sure to work for you. It has also been said that consuming 50 calories or less would not affect your intermittent process.

Doctors and scientists have agreed for years that the one true form of weight management is calorie restriction. Calorie restriction will work for you each and every time if you are able to stick with it. Most people who try calorie restricted diets often fall off the wagon because they are hungry all the time.

You will lose fat with this lifestyle, not because you're eating less, but because your're actually consuming the same amount of calories as if you didn't fast. The only difference is you consume all your calories in an 8-hour window. This process allows you the best of both worlds. You still get to eat all your favorite food while losing the weight you want. Although many people may prefer a burger with fries, having a healthy eating habit speeds up the process of loosing weight.

Despite the fact that you're eating every day on a calorie restricted diet, you usually don't care for what you're eating. Intermittent fasting however, gives you the control of what you are eating thus leaving you satisfied when you leave the dinner table. If you don't feel like you are dieting, you're more likely to stick with it.

Intermittent fasting involves alternating periods of feast and famine in which you may eat as much as you like during the feasting but drink only water during the fast. The aim is to achieve the benefits of calorie reduction and for some, use it as vehicle to lose weight.

Some of the things that may hinder your confidence in this lifestyle, is the fear that you will be extremely hungry and not be able to stick to the plan or do not know how to fit it into your schedule.

This is actually quite simple if you plan in advance you get eat your evening meal at pretty much the same time everyday but at an hour either side depending if on an intermittent fasting phase or an eating phase. Again with a little planning you can also accommodate socializing and eating out.

The main factor preventing many people from trying is the fear of being hungry. Although this does take a little will power and a slight degree of discomfort to begin with, it is actually quite easy.

Discover how to lose 30 pounds fast with intermittent fasting in this amazing book specially written just for you.

What are you waiting for? Let's get started.

CHAPTER 1

WHAT IS INTERMITTENT FASTING?

Intermittent Fasting (IF) refers to dietary eating patterns that involve not eating or severely restricting calories for a prolonged period of time. There are many different subgroups of intermittent fasting each with individual variation in the duration of the fast; some for hours, others for day(s).

This has become an extremely popular topic in the science community due to all of the potential benefits on fitness and health that are being discovered.

Fasting, or periods of voluntary abstinence from food has been practiced throughout the world for ages. Intermittent fasting with the goal of improving health is relatively new. Intermittent fasting involves restricting intake of food for a set period of time and does not include any changes to the actual foods you are eating.

Currently, the most common IF protocols are a daily 16 hour fast with an 8-hour eating window. Intermittent fasting could be considered a natural eating pattern that humans are built to implement and it traces all the way back to our paleolithic hunter-gatherer ancestors.

The current model of a planned program of intermittent fasting could potentially help improve many aspects of health from body composition to longevity and aging.

Although IF goes against the norms of our culture and common daily routine, the science may be pointing to less meal frequency and more time fasting as the optimal alternative to the normal breakfast, lunch, and dinner model.

Here are two common myths that pertain to intermittent fasting.

1 - You Must Eat 3 Meals Per Day: This "rule" that is common in Western society was not developed based on evidence for improved health, but was adopted as the common pattern for settlers and eventually became the norm. Not only is there a lack of scientific rationale in the 3 meal-a-day model, recent studies may be showing less meals and more fasting to be optimal for human health.

One study showed that one meal a day with the same amount of daily calories is better for weight loss and body composition than 3 meals per day. This finding is a basic concept that is extrapolated into intermittent fasting and those choosing to do IF may find it best to only eat 1-2 meals per day.

2 - You Need Breakfast, it's The Most Important Meal of The Day: Many false claims about the absolute need for a daily breakfast have been made. The most common claims being "breakfast increases your metabolism" and "breakfast decreases food intake later in the day".

These claims have been refuted and studied over a 16-week period with results showing that skipping breakfast did not decrease metabolism and it did not increase food intake at lunch and dinner.

It is still possible to do intermittent fasting protocols while still eating breakfast, but some people find it easier to eat a late breakfast or skip it altogether and this common myth should not get in the way.

Intermittent fasting is a controversial weight loss techni□ue because it involves not eating food for an extended period of time. Many people have the notion that not eating will slow down your metabolism and send your body into starvation mode, but it turns out this is not true at all.

In fact, the human body was designed to go long periods of time without eating, so intermittent fasting is actually a natural practice. Perhaps that is why it is so effective.

If you would like to lose weight but don't want to give up certain foods or don't want to partake in vigorous exercise, intermittent fasting is probably your best option. Fasting will help you lose weight □uickly, even if you don't eat extremely healthy or exercise, although that would greatly enhance your results.

This technique doesn't even require you to lower the amount of calories you consume. It simply takes a little bit of discipline in the beginning.

There are a few ways one can begin fasting. One method, the one I prefer, is daily fasting. This involves eating your food for the day within a time period of 6 to 8 hours. This would mean you fast for 16 to 18 hours every day.

The easiest way to do this is to skip breakfast in the mornings. You will benefit greatly from this. Even greater benefits will be experienced when you can lengthen the time spent fasting. For example, fast for 20 hours and eat for 4. Figure out what works best for you.

Another method that also works well is weekly fasting. This would involve a period of fasting that lasts between 24 and 36 hours. So, for example, you would eat as you normally do for 6 days of the week, then one day you would not eat any food at all.

Drink plenty of water during the time when you are not eating. Weekly fasting is also effective, but not as effective as daily fasting I have found. I encourage you to learn more and begin to incorporate one of these strategies into your life.

CHAPTER 2

TYPES OF INTERMITTENT FASTING

Intermittent fasting comes in various forms and each may have a specific set of unique benefits. Each form of intermittent fasting has variations in the fasting-to-eating ratio. The benefits and effectiveness of these different protocols may differ on an individual basis and it is important to determine which one is best for you.

Factors that may influence which one to choose include health goals, daily schedule/routine, and current health status. The most common types of IF are alternate day fasting, time-restricted feeding, and modified fasting.

1. ALTERNATE DAY FASTING:

This approach involves alternating days of absolutely no calories (from food or beverage) with days of free feeding and eating whatever you want.

This plan has been shown to help with weight loss, improve blood cholesterol and triglyceride (fat) levels, and improve markers for inflammation in the blood.

The main downfall with this form of intermittent fasting is that it is the most difficult to stick with because of the reported hunger during fasting days.

2. MODIFIED FASTING - 5:2 DIET

Modified fasting is a protocol with programmed fasting days, but the fasting days do allow for some food intake. Generally 20-25% of normal calories are allowed to be consumed on fasting days; so if you normally consume 2000 calories on regular eating days, you would be allowed 400-500 calories on fasting days.

The 5:2 part of this diet refers to the ratio of non-fasting to fasting days. So, on this regimen you would eat normally for 5 consecutive days, then fast or restrict calories to 20-25% for 2 consecutive days.

This protocol is great for weight loss, body composition, and may also benefit the regulation of blood sugar, lipids, and inflammation. Studies have shown the 5:2 protocol to be effective for weight loss, improve/lower inflammation markers in the blood (3), and show signs trending improvements in insulin resistance.

In animal studies, this modified fasting 5:2 diet resulted in decreased fat, decreased hunger hormones (leptin), and increased levels of a protein responsible for improvements in fat burning and blood sugar regulation (adiponectin).

The modified 5:2 fasting protocol is easy to follow and has a small number of negative side effects which included hunger, low energy, and some irritability when beginning the program.

Contrary to this however, studies have also noted improvements such as reduced tension, less anger, less fatigue, improvements in self-confidence, and a more positive mood

3. TIME-RESTRICTED FEEDING:

If you know anyone that has said they are doing intermittent fasting, odds are it is in the form of time-restricted feeding. This is a type of intermittent fasting that is used daily and it involves only consuming calories during a small portion of the day and fasting for the remainder.

Daily fasting intervals in time-restricted feeding may range from 12-20 hours, with the most common method being 16/8 (fasting for 16 hours, consuming calories for 8). For this protocol the time of day is not important as long as you are fasting for a consecutive period of time and only eating in your allowed time period.

For example, on a 16/8 time-restricted feeding program one person may eat their first meal at 7AM and last meal at 3PM (fast from 3PM-7AM), while another person may eat their first meal at 1PM and last meal at 9PM (fast from 9PM-1PM).

This protocol is meant to be performed every day over long periods of time and is very flexible as long as you are staying within the fasting/eating window(s).

Time-Restricted feeding is one of the most easy to follow methods of intermittent fasting. Using this along with your daily work and sleep schedule may help achieve optimal metabolic function. Time-restricted feeding is a great program to follow for weight loss and body composition improvements as well as some other overall health benefits.

The few human trials that were conducted noted significant reductions in weight, reductions in fasting blood glucose, and improvements in cholesterol with no changes in perceived tension, depression, anger, fatigue, or confusion.

Some other preliminary results from animal studies showed time restricted feeding to protect against obesity, high insulin levels, fatty liver disease, and inflammation.

The easy application and promising results of time-restricted feeding could possibly make it an excellent option for weight loss and chronic disease prevention/management. When implementing this protocol it may be good to begin with a lower fasting-to-eating ratio like 12/12 hours and eventually work your way up to 16/8 hours.

CHAPTER 3

BENEFITS OF INTERMITTENT FASTING SYSTEM

The diet you follow whilst Intermittent Fasting will be determined by the results that you are looking for and where you are starting out from as well, so take a look at yourself and ask the question what do I want from this?

If you are looking to lose a significant amount of weight then you are really going to have to take a look at your diet more closely, but if you just want to lose a few pounds for the beach then you may find that a few weeks of intermittent fasting can do that for you.

Although there are several different ways you can do intermittent fasting we are only going to look at the 16/8-hour fasting system which is what I used to lose 27 pounds over a 3 month period.

The basic method is to fast weekdays 16 hours a day, it makes sense to do this a few days apart and it is easier if you pick a day when you are busy so that you do not become distracted by feelings of hunger.

Initially you may feel some hunger pangs but these will pass and as you become more accustomed to intermittent fasting you may find as I have that feelings of hunger no longer present you with a problem. You may find that you have great focus and concentration whilst fasting which is the opposite of what you would expect but many people experience this.

Whilst fasting you can and should drink plenty of water to avoid dehydration, tea and coffee are okay as long as you only take a splash of milk.

If you are concerned that you are not getting enough nutrients into your body then you might consider a juice made from celery, broccoli, ginger and lime which will taste great and get some nutrient rich liquid into your body. Although if you can manage it then it would be best to stick to the water, tea and coffee.

Whatever your diet is whether it's healthy or not you should see weight loss after about 3 weeks of intermittent fasting and do not be discouraged if you don't notice much progress at first, it's not a race and it's better to lose weight in a linear fashion over time rather than crash losing a few pounds which you will put straight back on.

After the first month you may want to take a look at your diet on non-fasting days and cut out high sugar foods and any junk that you may normally eat. I have found that intermittent fasting over the long term tends to make me want to eat more healthy foods as a natural course.

If you are intermittent fasting for bodybuilding then you may want to consider looking at your macro nutrients and working out how much protein and carbohydrate you need to eat, this is much more complicated and you can find information about this on several websites which you will need to spend time researching for the best results.

There are many benefits to intermittent fasting which you will notice as you progress, some of these benefits include more energy, less bloating, a clearer mind and a general feeling of wellness. It's important not to succumb to any temptation to binge eat after a fasting period as this will negate the effect gained from the intermittent fasting period.

If you don't like the idea of fasting, perhaps the benefits will convince you to give it a try anyway. Intermittent fasting has many benefits that will greatly increase the □uality of your life. Some of the benefits include:

1. Improves Immune Function (Immune system booster)

The white blood cells of humans are an effective defense mechanism against pathogens in the body. However, white blood cells are limited by their ability to carry out their defensive function in entering cell and attacking intercellular pathogens.

This is because the primary line of defense of these pathogens are in fact lysosomes. Lysosomes through a process known as autophagy, which means self-eating, acts like the garbage disposal of the cell.

Damaged proteins, organelles, viruses, bacteria, and other pathogens are destroyed during autophagy. How long it is before your last meal directly impact lysosomal activities. Are you seeing the connection yet?

The function of lysosomes is to control the amount of nutrients that are available to the cells for the organelles to use. A filled stomach suppressed the functions of lysosomes and hence autophagy will not take place. Intermittent fasting allows the cells to undergo autophagy and hence lysosomes can carry out its garbage disposal function.

Autophagy is essential in destroying intercellular pathogens by restricting their source of nutrient. A dysfunction in autophagy at the cellular level can lead to all sorts of problem such as certain cancers, speeding up the aging process as well as neurological diseases.

2. Better Health

You benefit from a better, improve health from the fact that a properly functioning immune system provides a more robust defence against pathogen in the body. The only way to remain healthy is to develop a strong and robust immune system in your body.

Choosing one of the feeding windows in intermittent fasting well help to regulate insulin response and glycemic loads in the body. You have heard many, many times that many lifestyle diseases are the result of too much sugar in the blood stream. That is the blood sugar level is too high. Diseases such as obesity, and diabetes are all linked to this.

3. A superb way to burn excess fat during a workout

The whole purpose of aerobic endurance training is to burn unwanted fat. Health conscious gym adherent are on a constant look out for ways to burn fat. As such a high intensity exercise is one good way to cause the utilization of the body's fat storage instead of using glycogen.

By combining intermittent fasting and exercise you can increase fat utilization through ketosis. This is because your best fat burning work out is best done when your body is in a glycon depleted state.

These are just a few of the many benefits that fasting can offer you. If you simply want to be a healthier and/or happier person, it would be of your best interest to begin an intermittent fasting routine. So, how can you begin?

Intermittent fasting can add 40%-56% more years to your life. That in itself is reason enough to do it. However other benefits include body weight reduction and fat oxidation.

When you fast your body is forced to scavenge for fuel thus removing aged and damaged cells in the process. This sort of cleanses the body of undesirable and unwanted things and helps the weight loss and benefits of the good food choices be increased and more beneficial to your body.

Researchers are also saying that it might help age related deficits in cognitive function, too, so that tells me that it might help ward off Alzheimer's Disease and other types of Dementia.

Your risk of heart disease and other heart ailments may also be decreased when you start a healthy intermittent fasting regimen. Your risk for other chronic illnesses and diseases will also most likely be reduced.

A healthier you can begin with intermittent fasting and healthy food choices. Keep carbs to 50-100 grams per day. Many women eat between 1200-1500 calories per day, and when limiting their carbs, they are still losing weight. Men can handle up to 2000 calories per day. Of course less is best, and you need to determine caloric intake based on your activity such as working hard and exercising.

Drink lots of fluids, especially water and exercise in the evenings if possible. This will help with those late night cravings.

Once you start eating and drinking healthier, your body won't crave as much (if any) junk food, so making healthy food choices will simply get easier and easier as you progress in the intermittent fasting routine.

Alternate Day Fasting or ADF means alternating days of eating and not eating any food, but there is also an intermittent fasting called Modified Fasting where you consume about 20% of your normal calories one day and then eat normally (but healthy) the next day.

This is often more attainable for people because they feel less deprived when they are able to at least eat something daily, and it still has most of the benefits of the ADF regimen.

CHAPTER 4

HOW TO LOSE 30 POUNDS WITH INTERMITTENT FASTING

Intermittent fasting has become a popular way to use your body's natural fat-burning ability to lose fat in a short period of time. However, many people want to know, does intermittent fasting work and how exactly does it work?

When you go for an extended period of time without eating, your body changes the way that it produces hormones and enzymes, which can be beneficial for fat loss. These are the main fasting benefits and how they achieve those benefits.

Hormones form the basis of metabolic functions including the rate at which you burn fat. Growth hormone is produced by your body and promotes the breakdown of fat in the body to provide energy.

When you fast for a period of time, your body starts to increase its growth hormone production. Also, fasting works to decrease the amount of insulin present in the bloodstream, ensuring that your body burns fat instead of storing it.

A short term fast that lasts 12-72 hours increases the metabolism and adrenaline levels, causing you to increase the amount of calories burned. Additionally, people who fast also achieve greater energy through increased adrenaline, helping them to not feel tired even though they are not receiving calories generally.

Although you may feel as fasting should result in decreased energy, the body compensates for this, ensuring a high calorie burning regime.

Most people who eat every 3-5 hours primarily burn sugar instead of fat. Fasting for longer periods shifts your metabolism to burning fat. By the end of a 16-hour fast day, your body has used up glycogen stores in the first few hours and has spent of those hours burning through fat stores in the body.

For anyone who is regularly active, but still struggles with fat loss, intermittent fasting can help to increase fat loss without having to ramp up a workout regime or drastically alter a diet plan.

Another benefit of intermittent fasting is that it essentially resets a person's body. Going for a day or so without eating changes a person's craving, causing them to not feel as hungry over time.

If you struggle with constantly wanting food, intermittent fasting can help your body adjust to periods of not eating and help you to not feel hungry constantly. Many people notice that they begin to eat healthier and more controlled diets when they fast intermittently one day a week.

Intermittent fasting varies, but is generally recommended for about one day every week. During this day, a person may have water, tea or black coffee only.

As the body adjusts to an intermittent fasting regime, this usually is not necessary. Intermittent fasting helps to decrease fat stores naturally in the body, by switching the metabolism to break down fat instead of sugar or muscle.

It has been used by many people effectively and is an easy way to make a beneficial change. For anyone who struggles with stubborn fat and is tired of traditional dieting, intermittent fasting offers an easy and effective option for fat loss and a healthier lifestyle.

CHAPTER 5

WHAT MAKES INTERMITTENT FASTING DIFFERENT?

Intermittent fasting weight loss is one of the most effective ways to shed off your extra pounds. The ideas on intermittent fasting weight loss challenge most of the previously held beliefs on losing. Those who are seeking new ways to lose weight effectively have quickly embraced its ideas.

Let me start by clarifying that intermittent fasting is not a diet. You are probably tired of trying anything with the word 'diet' on it when it comes to weight loss. Intermittent fasting is a way of eating that involves a structured program on the times when you eat and when you do not eat.

You structure your program according to your fancy. If you can handle it, fast for a whole day. I recommend that you fast for 12 full hours before eating a meal. You can increase your fasting period later as you continue with the program.

What Makes it Different?

If you have tried to lose weight, you probably have tried diets such as Atkins diet based on the frequent feeding theory. Simply, proponents of such diets told you to eat often during the day. The idea was that the more you eat, the faster your metabolism.

The faster your metabolism, the more fat you will lose. Of course, you do know that the more you ate, the more you wanted to eat and the more your weight remained. When you are on an intermittent program, you will have to cut down your meal fre uency. Sometimes, you have to do without breakfast.

You probably sleep for around 6 to 8 hours. During this time, your body is in fasting mode. When your body is in fasting mode, it usually produces more insulin. More insulin in your body causes your body to have increased insulin sensitivity.

When your body has increased insulin sensitivity, you lose more fat. The brilliance of intermittent fasting weight loss program is that you skip breakfast to extend the period of your body's insulin sensitivity. This means that your body is going to be on fat loss mode for a longer period. You will lose more weight.

A longer fasting mode also has a good effect on the Growth hormone levels in your body. By skipping breakfast or eating during a specific period, your body produces Growth hormone. Growth hormone is what you want your body producing when you are trying to lose weight. This is simply because Growth hormone promotes weight loss in your body.

When you are on an intermittent fasting weight loss program, your Growth hormone levels are usually at their peak. You will be losing more weight during this period. High Growth hormone levels in your body also have several other health benefits. This program is simply amazing.

Intermittent fasting weight loss program is radically different from most weight loss programs being promoted in the market. However, its ideas are scientifically sound when it comes to losing weight. You should give this program a go if you are serious about weight loss.

CHAPTER 6

HOW TO DO INTERMITTENT FASTING

Intermittent fasting for beginners has two rules to follow: (1) Fasting has to be pleasurable and NOT stressful. (2) Fasting has to be simple and NOT rigid.

From an experienced faster's standpoint, I have a few suggestions for intermittent fasting beginners. There are two major reasons for people who want to do intermittent fasting (IF) - weight loss or health or both. In any case, it's good to observe these two formulas:

More rules = more complicated = low chance of success

Less rules = less complicated = high chance of success

In terms of health, a 16 hour period off of eating is very healthful, it helps you reduce calories without sacrificing what you like to eat on your non-fasting days, and maybe even more importantly it stimulates your body to produce more growth hormone.

Yes that's right growth hormone, the same one you hear about the celebrities taking to 'stay young'. Growth hormone has many anti-aging benefits, and one of the most interesting being fat burning.

There is no standard rule of doing IF. Simply try it and make it work for you. Let simplicity and flexibility be your fasting motto. Don't make it stressful for yourself.

As a beginner to practice intermittent fasting, I would say 'clear your mind from any other weight loss methods and focus on IF'. This is your first step towards IF success. Think how many times you've been told that breakfast is the most important meal in a day or you need to eat 6 to 10 small meals a day in order to lose weight.

I'm not saying these rules are wrong. If these rules work for you, stay with them. But if you are setting your feet onto the route of intermittent fasting, better put these concepts aside at least for the period you are trying out IF.

Having your IF mindset ready? Then begin with 'skip meal' and see how your body responds. I would say this is the simplest and easiest way to begin your intermittent fasting journey.

Pick a day to try 'skip breakfast'. Have black coffee, water or tea instead. If that works out fine, try 'skip lunch' and move on progressively. A 16-hour fast can be done by anybody with an appropriate fasting mindset. One useful tip is not to think of food. Avoid social talk at the pantry over lunch hour. Go out for a walk or do some simple exercises.

You can also explore these IF options:

• Condensed eating window, e.g. eat ONLY between 11am and 5pm;

• Skip meal on an unplanned basis, as far as it is natural and not interfere your daily work;

• Early and late, i.e. skip lunch;

• One meal a day, ideally dinner only when you are relaxed and really have time to enjoy food.

To repeat, fasting has to be pleasurable and not stressful. Don't press hard on yourself. Be flexible. This is very important.

CHAPTER 7

INTERMITTENT FASTING FOR BODYBUILDING

It is no secret that intermittent fasting helps rejuvenate the body and the fitness of a person, during intermittent fasting the person consumes only water, juices, or other low calorie substances. It signifies a period of eating followed by a period of non-eating.

However having water alone during the fasting helps to clean the body and drive out the impurities inside the body. In many cultures especially the Chinese intermittent fasting is more or less made compulsory to everyone, which enable people from those parts of the world to be highly agile and fit.

Fasting and bodybuilding are often related to each other, in order to build the body it is highly essential that the body be fit, for the body to be fit, one of the natural ways or the most effective way is intermittent fasting, as it helps in driving away the impurities of the body and gives the various organs that participate in the digestion of food their ☐uota of much needed rest.

Hence the person will start feeling more and more comfortable and happy with himself, this inbound feeling of wellness induces the confidence in the person and motivates him to build the body. Intermittent fasting bodybuilding hence is a natural way of improving ones fitness levels.

Points to be taken care of during intermittent fasting bodybuilding

1. For beginners the concept of intermittent fasting bodybuilding may seem to be a Herculean task, and may easily give up in no time, but it has to be understood that fasting at regular intervals of time helps oneself and boosts his confidence over a period of time. The perseverance has to be maintained in order to get the optimum results.

2. There is another tendency which we should be very wary of, and it is not to go overboard and strain yourself. Often people in a hurry to get fit and build the body of their dreams, fast too much that they fall sick, it should be avoided.

3. This can be avoided by keeping an eye out for the various hints and clues the body gives you. Like you should go and eat something and some food once you start feeling very giddy or a bit too tired or any other symbols that the body sends to indicate that its in dire need of some calories.

There is no point in fasting for a while and then shoving yourself with calories immediately after you have finished your fasting, instead slowly start taking in calories and exercise in the desired manner, making sure not to hurt yourself or overdo the exercises.

Fasting & bodybuilding are one of the oldest and the time tested methods of purifying one's own body and hence maintain it in proper condition. This helps you maintain your body in shape and also gives you the much needed confidence about yourself, above all it makes you realize the value of food and the importance of it.

Similarly it also forms one of the basic building blocks for body building, since for building a body it is essential that you have a conditioned body, if the body is not in a proper condition then it has to be brought to proper condition using the age old method of intermittent fasting and then build it.

CHAPTER 8

HOW TO DO IT HEALTHILY AND SAFELY

Intermittent fasting can improve health, reduce the risk of serious illness, and promote longevity. Perhaps you're intrigued and would like to give it a go but aren't sure how to start.

Or maybe you have tried it once or twice and found it too challenging. This chapter will give you strategies and guidelines to practice intermittent fasting safely and successfully.

There are three main ways to do intermittent fasting - a) only eat 8 hours a day and fast for 16 every day, b) a 24-hour fast on alternate days, or c) one or two 36-hour fasts each week.

It's worth experimenting with all 3 strategies to see which works best for you in terms of your lifestyle and effect on your health and wellbeing. The guidelines I've given you below are mainly for the 36hr fast, but most are helpful for the 24hr fast as well.

Pick a day that isn't too hectic or demanding because you may experience some detox reactions. Make sure you have the option to relax if you need to. You will get more out of the experience if you make time to turn inward, still the mind, meditate, contemplate, and listen to your inner guidance.

Enlist Support from people close to you before you start. It's great to fast with your partner so you can both motivate each other and share experiences.

Eat lightly the evening before by choosing a large salad or steamed vegetables with some lean protein. There is no point gorging the night before because it will make you feel even hungrier whilst you fast. It's best to avoid alcohol as well.

Keep hydrated during the fast as your body has an essential need for fluid. Water, herbal teas, are good choices. Have at least 2 litres of fluid during the day. Avoid fizzy drinks, fruit juice, and alcohol.

Have 1 or 2 glasses of vegetable juice as it will provide important electrolytes as well as having a health-boosting alkalizing effect. Try juicing celery, cucumber, chicory, fennel, and watercress. Avoid carrots and beets as they are □uite high in sugar.

Don't fight feeling hungry because you most probably will. Just be with the sensation without judgment, rather than resisting it (but read guideline 10 below).

Engage in light exercise such as walking, stretching, and gentle yoga. This is not the day to do an intense gym workout or anything too vigorous.

Add some breathing exercises such as yogic pranayama. A few minutes of practice offer amazing benefits from detoxification to boosting energy.

Expect some detox symptoms such as headaches, feeling groggy, or short periods of feeling jittery. These are made worse if you usually have lots of caffeine and sugar in your diet. Avoid taking over-the-counter medication to reduce these side effects. Instead rest, go for a walk, and practice breathing exercises.

Listen to your body wisdom and if you feel unwell or it gets too much then have some food. Your body knows best.

Break the fast gently the following morning. Have water or herb tea and a piece of fruit when you get up then 30min later have your usual breakfast. Eat as usual for the rest of the day (you probably won't feel the need to overeat).

Enjoy the changes in how you feel during and after the fast. Notice changes in your energy, emotions, and mental state. You may notice food is far more enjoyable on the day after the fast because your senses are heightened.

Recognize that it can take a few attempts to get used to this practice. After a few weeks your body will get used to it and the benefits you feel will increase as the discomfort simultaneously decreases.

Avoid intermittent fasting if you are pregnant, diabetic, suffering from a serious illness, or taking any prescribed medications. If in doubt it is best to consult with your health care provider.

CHAPTER 9

SECRETS OF SUCCESS WITH INTERMITTENT FASTING

Intermittent fasting is a method that, if used properly, can greatly enhance your health and increase your weight loss. "Fasting" is a term used to describe a period of time when you go without eating, as is common in some religious practices. The term "intermittent" refers to the alternation of periods of eating and of fasting.

So, intermittent fasting is basically a practice that involves eating within a certain time frame, and fasting in the time before and after. We all do this on a daily basis, since we are not eating when we are sleeping, but most of us do not "fast" for long enough periods of time to receive the benefits from it.

Let me explain how you can alter your way of eating so that you can lose weight extremely easily without changing the types of food you eat or the amount of calories you eat.

To get the most out of intermittent fasting, you need to fast for at least 16 hours. At 16 hours and above, some of the amazing benefits of intermittent fasting kick in. An easy way to do this is to simply skip breakfast every morning.

This is actually very healthy, but many people will try to tell you otherwise. By skipping breakfast, you are allowing your body to go into a caloric deficit, which will greatly increase the amount of fat you can burn and weight you can lose. Since your body is not busy digesting the food you ate, it has time to focus on burning your fat stores for energy and also for cleansing and detoxifying your body.

If you find it difficult to skip breakfast, you can instead skip dinner, although I find this much more difficult. It really does not matter, but the goal is to extend the period of time you spend fasting and decrease the amount of time you spend eating.

If you eat dinner at 6 o'clock at night, and don't eat until 10 the next morning, you have fasted for 16 hours. Longer is better, but you can see some pretty drastic changes from a daily 16 hour fast.

There are many ways to fast, and it is important that you choose the way that is best suited to your lifestyle so that you can stick with it and make it a lifetime habit. Above, I speak of a daily fast, but you can also do weekly, monthly or yearly fasts. All of them have many great benefits, and I encourage you to experience them for yourself.

Intermittent fasting may seem like a disastrous techni□ue to lose weight by starving the body, however in the reality it is not true. As the name implies, it is irregular starvation, not a regular one so the routine does more good than harm. It does not require one to eat sporadically, but the other way round.

This implies that a person may continue his or her usual eating routine, without having to do anything about the calorie intake. So if the diet comprises of bacon and eggs in the morning, a subway sandwich in the afternoon and a serving of lasagna in the evening, then this eating pattern does not have to break.

The only difference that will be observed will be a break of 16 hours in which the item to be consumed will be water. This fast is more or less like giving the digestive system a rest from fats, carbohydrates and proteins.

The idea is to not over work the body in the process of over consumption of food and less time to work it off through aerobic and anaerobic exercises, but giving the internal system a rest.

The best thing about this "rest" however, is that during this time span, the metabolism speeds up and also all the impurities are removed, as the only major consumption is of water.

In fact, it is not just the starvation of a day that does the magic, but rather the consumption of water that boosts up the results. Since the beginning of time, the advantages of water have been outlined. For every malady, the doctor stresses on the intake of water. Beauticians highlight the importance of water in keeping the skin free of acne and to keep the glow.

Dieticians stress on the intake of water. Even for aerobic and anaerobic exercises, the importance of having a good amount of water intake is stressed time and time again. So what spell does water basically cast on the body that makes it act like such a reliable agent?

As mentioned above, water speeds up the metabolism of the body. Since the kidneys need water to function properly and since most of the people out there have a low intake of water, it is up to the liver to make up for the loss of water.

This lowers the total output or the productivity of the liver. Since among other functions of the liver, the main one is to metabolize the fat stored, after performing the functions for the kidney, the liver is not able to metabolize the fat, therefore leading to an increase in the extra pounds mounting up on the figure.

The intermittent fast period of 16 hours, that can even exceed up to 36 hours depending on the will of the person, is a day dedicated to allowing the liver perform its functions without having to contribute to the chores of the kidneys due to the lack of water in the body.

This way, the body works more on the stored fats and burns them off effectively. So the rest from food day is primarily a day to boost up the metabolism to work off all the extra fat that the body has consumed due to lack of drinking ample water.

Another advantage that intermittent fasting has for the body, apart from speeding up the metabolism is that of helping lose all the water weight stored in the body. How the water got stored in the hips, thighs, legs and stomach is primarily due to an inconsistent flow of water.

The body stored all the water since it was not receiving the re□uired amount daily. Therefore, once the supply of water is plentiful, the body automatically decides to let go of all the water stored in the shape of fat and drastically cuts down the body weight.

Furthermore, with ample intake of water, it has been observed that the body starts to re□uire a less food. Therefore, during the intermittent fasting time span as the body consumes a vast □uantity of water, there is less craving for food items as it appears that the stomach is well nourished.

In accordance with that, water also helps to preserve the muscle mass, allowing better work outs. So if during your intermittent fast you aim to take a walk for 45 minutes or get up on the treadmill, keeping yourself well hydrated is the key solution to feeling fresh even after the work out.

Intermittent fasting is indeed the best way to work towards a consistent weight loss program. The results however will not be immediate but there will not be a time period, of even a week, when a loss of 1lb does not show on the scale. Adopting this ritual is a smart technique towards smart weight loss.

CHAPTER 10

INTERMITTENT FASTING TO COMPLEMENT YOUR WEIGHT LOSS EXERCISES

Food is important but occasional fasting is also a great idea, if losing weight is your goal. Experts agree that intermittent fasting is an ideal way through which a restriction on calories can be imposed to scoop out beneficial effects from a weight loss exercise routine.

Just skipping a meal is not what it implies. Putting your body on a fast for approximately 12 hours or more is technically termed as intermittent fasting. Body weight trainers agree that this is fast becoming a popular option with all classes of people who target substantial weight loss in a short period of time.

Your basal metabolic rate, more popularly known as BMR can be an effective guide to the amount of calories that you need to keep your system running. Entering your weight, age and height in a BMR calculator can pop up the result fast and smooth. This way, you get a comprehensive idea of your daily calorie re□uirements.

Understanding this is important as intermittent fasting must be followed by a diet plan which is chalked out as per the shown result. Gorging on endless calories when you resume eating can make your efforts go down the drain.

A fasting for two days per week (not simultaneous) and a sensible eating plan thereafter, punctuated by supervised bodyweight exercise routines is the ideal key to a healthy weight loss plan.

If you are worrying about energy and how you would cope up without food for so long, then don't panic and just relax. Studies have shown that intermittent fasting not only improves your energy quotient but also fuels up your metabolism, two things every trainer vouches on for effective results. It is hugely different from traditional modes of fasting which often leave you dizzy and drained.

Fractional calorie elimination has been seen to give rise to depression and high irritability in humans. Rather than cutting calories from regular diet portions, a complete intermittent fasting can eliminate the problems that usually tags with other kinds of fasting. This can not only pep up your energy levels but also bring to you a host of benefits.

Among the most obvious benefits come a cut on increased blood pressure, a check on diabetes, enhanced longevity, lowered stress levels and a feel good factor, not to mention significant weight loss in a short time.

When starting a fasting program like this, do ensure that you make a slow beginning, like fasting for a single day in a week until your body is ready to accept a fasting period for two days.

Design your bodyweight exercise schedules in a suitable fashion during this period, preferably at a moderate pace, until your body is capable to take a fully loaded exercise routine. As you get used to it, the results start showing on your body in a positive way.

CHAPTER 11

AMAZING TRUTHS ABOUT INTERMITTENT FASTING

If you have ever struggled to lose weight or have actually managed to suffer enough to lose a bit of weight only to see it come straight back (plus more.) afterward, you are probably wondering if any diet approach can work. Perhaps it is time you considered intermittent fasting.

Although fasting has been around for thousands of years, it is only recently that the advantages of intermittent fasting for fat-loss have really been explored. So what is intermittent fasting?

Basically, this involves alternating periods of fasting with an eating window. These periods can be daily. For example a 16 hour daily fast. Another possibility is doing a 24 hour fast once or twice a week. Both approaches work well and will help shed stubborn body fat

Let me share some amazing truths about intermittent fasting

1. You won't feel nearly as hungry as you think you will. In fact, I have found that I don't think any more about food than I normally do. The first time I tried it I was a bit wary, but I found it to be wonderfully easy.

2. Your concentration levels will improve dramatically. If I have a particularly technical piece of work to do, then I save it for one of my fast days as I know that I will be able to focus on it far more effectively.

3. You save money. It's an obvious benefit really - you don't pay for food you don't eat. When I was on a six small meals a day regime, I used to have to do a supermarket shop just to get all my food for the week organized. I am free from that now.

4. The weight will fall off you like crazy. I have been amazed at just how quickly the excess pounds have been shed, and continue to go. The last two months included Christmas, and I love my food and drink, and I still came out of it slimmer than when I went in. Losing weight quickly is a formality.

5. You will feel happier. You are on the path to the body that you deserve and each passing week will show you the progress that you are making. It is really motivational and empowering.

6. Nothing else in your life need change. Here's a typical Sunday for me: sandwich for breakfast, two pints in my local at lunchtime, roast lamb/beef dinner, a few glasses of wine, then in the evening a light snack. I have done this every Sunday since I started intermittent fasting just to remind myself that I can and should still enjoy life's pleasures.

7. You have more time. I've noticed that I have at least an hour extra productive time on my fast days simply because I am not preparing or cooking food, or clearing up afterwards.

8. Great sleep. I sleep like a baby on my fast days. Probably because I am not so full of food.

9. Way more energy. I feel like I am ten years younger. This might be because I am so much lighter, but it might be more to do with my blood sugar levels regulating better, which is a beneficial side effect of intermittent fasting.

10. Compulsive eating is massively reduced. I seem to have lost the desire to eat crisps, snacks and other diet minefields. It is as though intermittent fasting resets the way you eat.

11. You can make it a part of your life, overnight. By the time I had completed my second fast, I knew that I could make intermittent fasting an integral part of my routine. And, by so doing, the weight loss that I wanted so badly would happen automatically.

12. No tiny ready meals or snack bars. I just can't be doing with all the milkshakes and snack bars that the large diet companies think are going to satisfy me. I want to eat real food in normal portions.

13. Eat when you want. Don't do breakfast? No worries. It's overrated anyway. Don't want to eat little and often? No problem. Just eat like you normally would, and do one or two twenty-four hour fasts per week. Or if you want to make it part of your lifestyle, do the 16/8 method daily.

14. Gain confidence. As you get slimmer and fit your clothes better - and buy yourself some new ones - you can't help but feel increased self-assurance.

CHAPTER 12

QUESTIONS ABOUT INTERMITTENT FASTING AND SUPPLEMENTS

At bare minimum, everyone should be taking a multivitamin of some sort because of nutrient deficient soil. I prefer organic, whole food vitamin sources such as powdered greens.

What supplements should I be taking?

A multivitamin, an omega 3 source, a probiotic, and Vitamin D. As I said before, I prefer whole food sources over artificial multivitamins. So I would use a greens source as my multivitamin. I use a high quality fish oil or krill oil for my omega 3 source.

An alternative for vegans would be flaxseed oil or hemp oil. As for probiotics, the best source is naturally fermented foods such as miso soup, kimchi, natto, kefir, and sauerkraut.

As for supplementation, get one that has more than 10 billion active probiotic strains per serving. Vitamin D supplementation is very important for people who don't get one hour of sunlight exposure per day.

For instance, if you live in the northeast US, you will definitely need it. People with darker complexions will need more sun exposure than light skinned folks because UV-B rays do not penetrate the skin as far. Therefore, less sunlight is converted to Vitamin D. The latest studies are saying that almost everyone is deficient in Vitamin D.

What is the best type of protein powder to buy?

It depends on what you are using it for. Whey is the best all-purpose protein. It absorbs fast, is cheap, and is best taken after a workout. Casein protein is best taken before bed because it is slowly absorbed. I would stick to a protein powder that is made from grass-fed cow's milk for higher quality.

When should I take my protein supplement: before or after a workout?

If you can afford it, both. The influx of branch chained amino acids taken before will give you a better performance throughout your workout. If you are trying to save money, the optimal time to take a protein supplement is within 30 minutes of completing your workout for recovery.

What's the easiest way to see results without dieting?

Intermittent fasting may work for you. Research shows that the 18th hour is the "golden hour". This is when you see the most results for the least amount of time. There are different theories on intermittent fasting. Some say the fast starts after your last meal and others say that it starts 2 or 3 hours after your last meal due to digestion.

CONCLUSION

Intermittent fasting is a feeding pattern which alternates between periods of fasting and controlled eating. It is a simple dietary method divided into many types.

One of the intermittent fasting methods is alternate day fasting, whereby a person takes a normal diet on particular days of the week and fasts on some. During the fasting days, one does not fully abstain from food but rather reduces calorie intake to 1/4 of the normal diet.

The other fasting type is whereby eating is restricted to a certain time window within a day. This means restricting eating between an 8 hour window eating period, which means a person eats once in every eight hours.

Some people however reduce the span to either six, four or even two hours according to their convenience. The longest time that a person can stay without food on intermittent fasting is 36 hours. If practiced accordingly, it can result in a number of positive health effects.

For instance, intermittent fasting promotes general good health. It significantly reduces cravings for snack foods and sugars. The practice normalizes insulin as well as leptin sensitivity. Insulin resistance contributes to many chronic diseases such as diabetes, cancer and heart infections. Intermittent fasting will therefore protect the body from such infections.

Intermittent fasting results in improved brain health. Fasting helps the body to convert stored glycogen into glucose to release energy. If the fasting proceeds for some time, continued breakdown of body fats induces the liver to secrete ketone bodies.

These small molecules are by-products of fatty acids synthesis, and the brain can use them as fuel. Research also indicates that exercise and fasting results in genes and other growth factors which are essential in recycling and rejuvenating the brain.

This type of fasting also boosts body fitness and loss of weight. Combined fasting and exercise increases effects of catalysts and cellular factors so that breakdown of glycogen and fats is maximized. Exercising while hungry therefore forces the body to burn stored fats for significant weight loss.

The program is also known to prevent cognitive decline. Research was conducted in 2006 on mice, in which water maze tests were used to assess cognitive functions of mice on normal diet and those on intermittent fasting. It was discovered that mice put on intermittent fasting experienced slower cognitive declines, which too applies to human beings.

Intermittent fasting will also boost muscle building especially in men. This is because after eating, the energy gained will be used to sustain a workout session.

But if training is done while fasting, the body utilizes stored body fats to sustain the exercises. Eating after the session ensures that the energy gained is utilized in replenishing the body in the best way. This assists the muscles to □uickly recover and build up.

In conclusion, intermittent fasting is a healthy practice but requires discipline to maintain the benefits. In essence less is more, the more you fast the more you can eat in your 8-hour window. It might not be the easiest thing you do, but once you see results it will be worth it. You will need commitment and perseverance to move through the changes in diet, since only consistency will achieve these positive results. It changed my life and helped me to lose weight, feel great and save money as well. I am blessed to share my knowlege with you

Thanks for reading.